Gauri Eknath Solanke

The Blue Pea Plant

Gauri Eknath Solanke

The Blue Pea Plant

The wonders of Clitoria Ternatea

LAP LAMBERT Academic Publishing

Imprint

Cover image: www.ingimage.com

Publisher:
LAP LAMBERT Academic Publishing
is a trademark of
Dodo Books Indian Ocean Ltd. and OmniScriptum S.R.L publishing group

120 High Road, East Finchley, London, N2 9ED, United Kingdom
Str. Armeneasca 28/1, office 1, Chisinau MD-2012, Republic of Moldova, Europe
Managing Directors: Ieva Konstantinova, Victoria Ursu
info@omniscriptum.com

Printed at: see last page
ISBN: 978-620-8-47492-8

Gauri E. Solanke

The Blue Pea Plant : Wonders of the Clitoria Ternatea

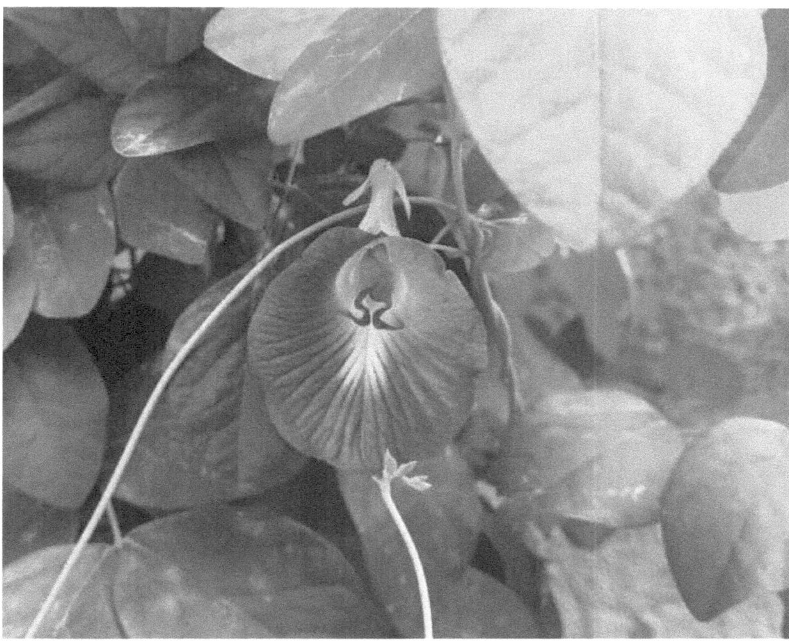

PHARMACOGNOSY : BOOK ON THE BLUE PLANT

Gauri E. Solanke

Miss. Gauri E. Solanke

B. Pharmacy

Pravara Rural College Of Pharmacy

Loni – 413736

E – Mail – gaurisolanke7@gmail.com

Table of Contents

Chapter 1: Introduction :-

1.1 Overview

Clitoria ternatea, commonly known as the butterfly pea, is a herbaceous plant celebrated not only for its stunning deep blue flowers but also for its extensive medicinal, agricultural, and ornamental value. Belonging to the family Fabaceae (Leguminosae), this plant is widely distributed in tropical and subtropical regions across Asia, Africa, and parts of South America.

Traditionally used in Ayurvedic, Siddha, and Chinese medicine, Clitoria ternatea has gained attention in recent decades due to the discovery of its neuroprotective, antioxidant, anxiolytic, anti-inflammatory, anti-cancer, and antimicrobial properties. The plant's utility is further enhanced by its role in sustainable agriculture, where it is used as a nitrogen-fixing cover crop.

The plant's striking blue petals contain anthocyanin compounds (especially ternatins) that are pH-sensitive and used as natural food colorants and indicators in chemistry, as well as in the cosmetic and wellness industry. The flowers are also used to prepare vibrant herbal teas, which have become increasingly popular worldwide.

1.2 Taxonomical Classification

Category	Classification
Kingdom	Plantae
Subkingdom	Tracheobionta
Division	Magnoliophyte

Class	Magnoliopsida
Order	Fabales .
Family	Fabaceae (Leguminosae)
Genus	Clitoria
Species	Clitoria ternatea L.

1.3 Etymology and Botanical Name

The genus name "Clitoria" was coined by 17th century botanist Carl Linnaeus, inspired by the flower's shape.

It's petals said to resemble the human female clitoris, drawing upon ancient symbolic interpretations of the flower representing femininity, fertility, and purity. Because of this it has historically been considered a plant with aphrodisiac qualities in some cultures.

The species epithet "ternatea" is derived from the island of Ternate in Indonesia which was also known as "Maluku Island", where the plant was first documented by European botanists.

1.4 Common Names

The plant is often associated with purity, protection and spiritual significance in India and Southeast Asia. In various different regions known by different names.

Language	**Common Name**
English	Butterfly pea, Blue pea, Asian pigeonwings, Cordofan pea
Sanskrit	Vishnukranta, Aparajita
Marathi	Gokarna

Hindi	Aparajita
Bengali	Aparajita
Malayalam	Shankupushpam
Telugu	Sankhu Poolu
Tamil	Sangu Poo
Indonesian	Bunga Telang
Thai	Dok Anchan

1.5 Historical and Cultural Significance

Clitoria ternatea holds a sacred place in many cultures, particularly in India, where it is associated with spiritual purity and devotion. It is traditionally offered to deities such as Lord Shiva and Goddess Durga during religious rituals.

In Ayurvedic texts, the plant is known as "Medhya Rasayana" (Brain tonic), a rejuvenator for the brain and nervous system. In Unani medicine, it is valued for it's diuretic, laxative and anti-inflammatory effects. It has been used historically to treat a variety of conditions including:

Memory loss and cognitive decline

Epilepsy and mental disorder

Infections and fevers

Infertility and menstrual disorders

In Southeast Asia, the flowers are used to make a blue-colored drink known as "Nam Dok Anchan" in Thailand, or mixed with lemon to produce a purple hue - a natural pH indicator effect used in food and beverages.

1.6 Geographical Distribution

The species epithet ternatea comes from Ternate Island (Indonesia), where it was first described. It is believed to be native to tropical Asia, particularly the Indian subcontinent ans Southeast Asia.

It thrives in tropical and subtropical climates. It requires warm temperatures (20–30°C) and is frost sensitive.

Specially found in roadsides, gardens, grasslands, forest edges and agricultural fields. Commonly, it is cultivated in home gardens for it's flowers and medicinal use.

Clitoria ternatea is now naturalized across tropical and subtropical regions globally, including:

India

Thailand

Indonesia

Malaysia

Sri Lanka

Africa

Central and South America

Australia

1.7 Botanical Importance

Clitoria ternatea, commonly known as the butterfly pea, holds significant botanical importance as a member of the family Fabaceae. Like other legumes, it possesses the unique ability to fix atmospheric nitrogen through symbiotic association with Rhizobium bacteria present in its root nodules. This not only enriches soil fertility but also makes the plant valuable in crop rotation, green manuring, and sustainable agriculture.

Morphologically, the plant is a perennial twining herb characterized by its typical papilionaceous flowers, which display vibrant shades of blue, purple, or white. The distinct floral structure makes it an important species for studying pollination biology within the Fabaceae. Its flowers are insect-pollinated, primarily by bees and butterflies, thereby contributing to the maintenance of biodiversity and serving as a nectar source for pollinators.

Botanically, the plant is also valued for its phytochemical composition, particularly the presence of rare polyacylated anthocyanins called ternatins, which impart the intense blue color to the flowers. These compounds, along with flavonoids and saponins, have attracted interest in the fields of pharmacognosy, phytochemistry, and natural dye research.

Additionally, Clitoria ternatea serves an ornamental role due to its striking flowers and rapid growth habit, making it a popular climber in gardens and landscapes. Agriculturally, it is used as fodder for livestock owing to its high protein content and drought tolerance, which allows its cultivation in semi-arid regions.

Thus, in botanical terms, Clitoria ternatea is significant as a nitrogen-fixing legume, a pollinator-friendly species, a phytochemically rich plant, and an agriculturally beneficial crop, reflecting its wide ecological and scientific value.

1.8 Economic and Industrial Relevance

The economic potential of Clitoria ternatea has increased considerably in recent years due to its:

Use as a natural food and beverage colorant

Application in cosmetic products (anti-aging, skin tone enhancers)

Inclusion in herbal supplements for brain health and immunity

Potential role in pharmaceutical formulations

Use as a bioindicator and dye in textile industries

Its low toxicity and rich phytochemical profile make it a promising candidate for commercialization in herbal and wellness industries.

1.9 Need for Scientific Exploration

Despite centuries of traditional use, Clitoria ternatea remains understudied in terms of large-scale clinical trials, biotechnology applications, and pharmacogenomic research.

However, initial studies have shown promising effects in neuroprotection, memory enhancement, diabetes management, and cancer inhibition.

Studying this plant not only supports the advancement of ethnopharmacology and herbal drug development, but also encourages sustainable agriculture and eco-friendly product development.

Chapter 2: Botanical Description :-

2.1 General Morphology

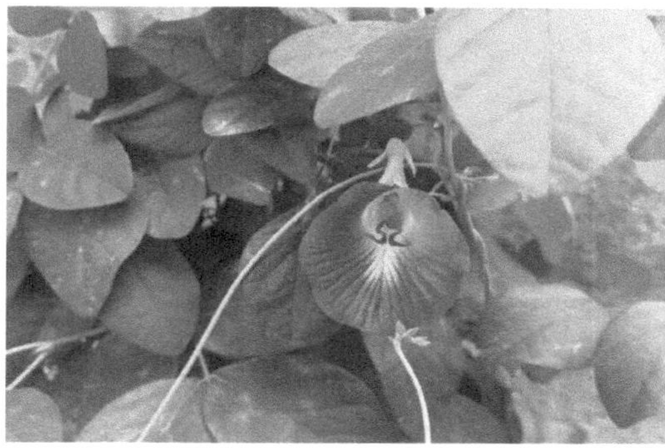

Clitoria ternatea is a perennial, herbaceous climbing vine that is both hardy and adaptive to various soil and climate conditions.

It exhibits typical characteristics of the Fabaceae family, with compound leaves and papilionaceous (butterfly-shaped) flowers.

The plant can grow as a trailing creeper or a twining climber, often supported by trellises, fences, or other plants.

2.1.1 Root System

Type: Taproot system

The roots are long, thick, and fibrous, allowing the plant to penetrate deep into the soil.

Root nodules are present, housing nitrogen-fixing Rhizobium bacteria, which enhance soil fertility by converting atmospheric nitrogen into usable forms for plants.

2.1.2 Stem

The stem is slender, green, and soft in young plants, turning woody at the base with age.

It is twining and weakly climbing, relying on support for vertical growth.

Internodes are long, and branches often grow profusely under favorable conditions.

2.1.3 Leaves

Type: Pinnately compound

Each leaf typically has 5 to 7 obovate leaflets arranged oppositely along a central rachis.

Leaflets: Smooth, green, ovate to elliptical, about 3–5 cm long.

The leaves are glabrous (smooth) with a prominent midrib and reticulate venation.

Stipules are small and deciduous.

2.1.4 Flower

Type: Papilionaceous (typical of Fabaceae), complete, bisexual, and zygomorphic.

Color: Most commonly deep blue with yellow markings on the throat, but white and light purple varieties also exist.

Size: Approximately 4–6 cm in diameter.

Shape: The flower consists of five petals—standard (banner), wings, and keel (fused lower petals).

Arrangement: Solitary, axillary flowers borne on short peduncles.

Blooming pattern: Flowers open in the early morning and fade by evening; blooming occurs throughout the year in tropical regions.

Pollination: Primarily by insects (entomophily), especially bees.

2.1.5 Fruit

Type: Linear pod (legume).

Size: 5–7 cm long, flat, slightly curved.

Color: Green when young, turning brown and woody when mature.

Dehiscence: The mature pod splits open longitudinally to release seeds. Each pod contains 6–10 flattened seeds.

2.1.6 Seeds

Color: Brown to gray.

Shape: Flattened and elliptical.

Size: Small, about 5–7 mm.

Germination: Seeds exhibit hard seed coats and may require scarification or soaking in water to enhance germination rate.

2.2 Varieties and Flower Colors

Clitoria ternatea has several natural and cultivated varieties, mostly categorized based on flower color and number of petals:

Variety	Flower Color	Description
Single Blue	Deep blue	Most common, with yellow markings
Double Blue	Deep blue	More petals, ornamental use
Single White	Pure white	Medicinal and spiritual use
Double White	White	Rare, ornamental and religious use

Purple or Lavender	Light purple	Less common, hybrid varieties

The blue-flowered single petal variety is the most pharmacologically studied due to its high anthocyanin (ternatin) content.

2.3 Microscopic Features (Powdered Drug Analysis)

For pharmacognostical evaluation, the plant parts (especially flower and root) show the following microscopic features when powdered:

1) Trichomes: Unicellular, non-glandular, often present in the leaf and calyx.
2) Starch grains: Rounded, seen in root and stem sections.
3) Calcium oxalate crystals: Found in parenchyma cells.
4) Vessels and fibers: Lignified, visible in stem and root powder.
5) Pollen grains: Round, with spiny exine, observed in flower powder.

2.4 Photoperiod and Environmental Adaptations

1. Photoperiod Sensitivity

Clitoria ternatea is a short-day plant, meaning it flowers when the length of daylight is shorter than a critical threshold.

Flower initiation is regulated by the phytochrome system, which senses changes in day length.

Under long-day conditions, the plant tends to remain vegetative longer, with delayed flowering.

2. Temperature Adaptations

Thrives best in warm tropical and subtropical climates (20–30°C).

Sensitive to frost and extreme cold, which can damage roots and inhibit flowering.

Tolerates moderately high temperatures up to 35–37°C but requires adequate soil moisture.

3. Soil and Moisture Requirements

Adapted to a wide range of soils (sandy loam to clay), but prefers well-drained, fertile soils with neutral to slightly acidic pH (6.0–7.5).

Drought-tolerant due to its deep root system, but optimal growth is observed under moderate irrigation.

Sensitive to waterlogging, which may cause root rot.

4. Light Intensity

Requires full sunlight for vigorous growth and maximum flower production.

Shaded conditions lead to reduced flowering and lower anthocyanin content in petals.

5. Ecological Significance

Its ability to adapt to various climates makes it a valuable cover crop and green manure in agriculture.

Plays a role in soil nitrogen fixation through its root nodules, enhancing soil fertility.

6. Watering: Drought-tolerant but prefers moderate watering during flowering phase.

2.5 Growth and Lifespan

Growth rate: Fast-growing; flowers may appear within 6–8 weeks of sowing.

Life span: Clitoria ternatea is a long-lived perennial under favorable conditions, with a lifespan of 2–3 years or more.

In cultivation, it is often treated as an annual or biennial for higher yield and ease of management.

The plant regenerates each year from its deep rootstock, even after periods of drought or pruning.

Flowering season: Nearly year-round in warm climates, with peak blooming in summer and monsoon seasons.

2.6 Ecological Role

1.It helps in fixing atmospheric nitrogen into the soil, improving fertility and reducing the need for chemical fertilizers. It is often used in crop rotation and intercropping to enhance soil quality.

2. Its vibrant blue (sometimes white) flowers attract a wide range of pollinators like bees, butterflies, and other insects. This supports biodiversity and helps maintain healthy pollinator populations in ecosystems.

3. The plant is rich in protein and serves as nutritious fodder for cattle, goats, and other livestock. This contributes to the food chain and sustainable livestock farming.

4. Clitoria ternatea has a creeping/climbing growth habit with dense foliage. It provides ground cover, reduces soil erosion, and improves moisture retention in degraded or semi-arid lands.

Chapter 3: Cultivation and Propagation

3.1 Introduction

Clitoria ternatea is a low-maintenance, fast-growing perennial herbaceous plant that thrives in warm climates.

Its ability to grow in varied environmental conditions, along with its agronomic and medicinal value, makes it a suitable crop for home gardens, commercial cultivation, and intercropping systems.

Additionally, its capacity to fix atmospheric nitrogen enhances soil fertility, making it a valuable green manure plant.

This chapter discusses the agronomic practices, propagation techniques, optimal conditions, and plant protection measures required for the successful cultivation of Clitoria ternatea.

3.2 Climatic Requirements

Climate: Tropical and subtropical

1. Temperature: Thrives best in warm tropical and subtropical climates.

Optimum growth occurs between 20–30°C.

Can tolerate temperatures up to 35–37°C if soil moisture is adequate.

Frost-sensitive – prolonged cold can damage shoots and roots, reducing flowering and survival.

2. Rainfall: Requires moderate rainfall (700–1500 mm annually) for ideal growth.

Well-adapted to both monsoon climates and areas with distinct wet and dry seasons.

Drought tolerance is enhanced by its deep root system, but prolonged drought reduces flower and seed yield.

Waterlogging is harmful and should be avoided.

3. Light: A sun-loving plant, requiring full sunlight (6–8 hours daily) for maximum photosynthesis and flower production.

Shaded environments lead to weak growth and reduced flowering.

4. Humidity: Performs well in moderate to high humidity (50–80%), which supports lush vegetative growth.

Extremely dry air can cause flower and leaf drop.

5. Altitude: Best adapted to lowland and mid-altitude regions (up to ~1500 m above sea level).

Growth is slower at higher altitudes due to lower temperatures.

6. Seasonal Suitability: In tropical climates: Can flower year-round, with peak blooming in post-monsoon to autumn.

In subtropical regions: Flowering is seasonal, strongly influenced by day length (photoperiod) and temperature.

7. Agricultural Significance: Its wide adaptability makes it suitable as Ornamental plant in gardens (for flowers).

Forage and cover crop in tropical agriculture.

Green manure to improve soil fertility in regions with varying climate conditions.

3.3 Soil Requirements

Type: Well-drained loamy or sandy-loam soils

pH: 6.0 to 7.5 (neutral to slightly acidic)

Drainage: Proper drainage is essential to prevent root rot

Fertility: Though it can thrive in low-fertility soils due to nitrogen fixation, yield improves with organic compost application.

3.4 Land Preparation

1. Ploughing: The land should be ploughed 2–3 times to a fine tilth.

2. Bed Formation: Raised beds can be used in areas with heavy rainfall to improve drainage.

3. Soil Enrichment: Application of well-rotted farmyard manure (FYM) at 8–10 tons/acre improves soil texture and fertility.

4. Biofertilizers: Rhizobium and phosphate-solubilizing bacteria may be inoculated to enhance root nodulation and growth.

3.5 Propagation Methods

3.5.1 By Seeds (Most Common)

Seed Treatment: Seeds have a hard seed coat; soaking in warm water (40–50°C) for 6–8 hours or scarification using sandpaper improves germination.

Sowing Time: Best during the onset of monsoon (June–July) or early spring (Feb–March) in irrigated conditions.

Spacing: Row to row: 60 cm

Plant to plant: 30 cm

Seed Rate: Approximately 5–6 kg/acre.

3.5.2 By Stem Cuttings (Less Common)

Cuttings: 15–20 cm long healthy, mature stems with 2–3 nodes

Rooting: Can be rooted in soil, water, or sand with light moisture

Rooting Hormones: Application of IBA (Indole-3-butyric acid) improves root initiation

This method is used primarily for preserving specific flower color traits (e.g., double white variety).

3.6 Germination and Seedling Management

Germination Period: 7–12 days

Transplantation: Seedlings can be transplanted after 3–4 weeks when they reach 10–15 cm height

Mulching: Mulching with straw or dry leaves helps retain moisture and suppress weeds.

3.7 Fertilizer and Nutrient Management

Organic Fertilizers: 10–15 tons/ha of compost or FYM during land preparation

Inorganic Fertilizers (if needed):

Nitrogen: 20 kg/ha

Phosphorus: 40 kg/ha

Potassium: 20 kg/ha

Micronutrients: Foliar spray of seaweed extract or micronutrient mix during the vegetative stage can enhance flowering.

3.8 Irrigation Management

Frequency: During germination: every 2–3 days

After establishment: once a week or as required

Overwatering should be avoided to prevent fungal infections and root diseases

Drip irrigation is ideal for water conservation and uniform application.

3.9 Support and Trellising

Although Clitoria ternatea can grow as a bushy plant, climbing varieties need support

Use bamboo stakes, trellises, or wire mesh to guide vertical growth

Trellising improves flower visibility and harvesting ease.

3.10 Intercropping and Companion Planting

Often used as a cover crop or green manure in orchards and vegetable gardens

Can be intercropped with:

Banana

Papaya

Turmeric

Legumes (groundnut, soybean)

3.11 Pest and Disease Management

3.11.1 Common Pests

Pest	Symptoms	Control
Aphids	Curling yellowing of leaves	Neem oil spray or insecticidal soap
Leaf miners	Tunnels inside leaves	Pruning affected parts, neem extract
Caterpillars	Eat leaves and buds	Manual removal or Bt (Bacillus thuringiensis) spray

3.11.2 Common Diseases

Disease	Symptoms	Control
Powdery mildew	White powdery spots on leaves	Sulfur-based fungicides, good air circulation
Root rot	Wilting, blackened roots	Avoid waterlogging, use Trichoderma in soil

3.12 Harvesting

Flower Harvesting:

Flowers should be picked early in the morning when fully bloomed.

Harvesting is done manually, and frequent plucking encourages more blooming.

Seed Harvesting:

Allow pods to mature and dry on the plant before collecting.

Seeds are separated, dried, and stored in airtight containers.

3.13 Post-Harvest Handling

Fresh flowers should be used or processed immediately.

Drying: Flowers can be shade-dried at 30–35°C and stored for up to 6 months.

Storage: Store in airtight, moisture-proof containers to retain color and potency.

Seeds: Can remain viable for 1–2 years when stored in cool, dry conditions.

3.14 Yield

Fresh flowers: 1–1.5 tons per acre per year (depending on variety and conditions).

Dried flowers: 250–300 kg per acre.

Seeds: 100–150 kg/acre.

Chapter 4: Phytochemical Constituents

4.1 Introduction

Clitoria ternatea has emerged as a plant of considerable pharmacological interest, largely due to its rich and diverse phytochemical profile.

Various parts of the plant—including the roots, stems, leaves, flowers, and seeds—contain biologically active compounds responsible for its traditional and modern therapeutic uses.

Among its most remarkable compounds are anthocyanins, flavonoids, alkaloids, saponins, and triterpenoids, many of which contribute to the plant's nootropic, antioxidant, anti-inflammatory, and antimicrobial activities.

This chapter details the phytochemicals identified in Clitoria ternatea, their distribution in plant parts, and their medicinal relevance.

4.2 Major Chemical Constituents

The key classes of phytochemicals in Clitoria ternatea include:

Class of Compound	Notable Examples
Anthocyanins	Ternatins A1, A2, B1, B2, D1, D2, E, F
Flavonoids	Kaempferol, Quercetin, Myricetin, Delphinidin
Triterpenoids	Taraxerol, Taraxerone
Alkaloids	Clitorine
Saponins	Clitoriaside A, Clitoriaside B
Steroids	Beta-sitosterol
Phenolic compounds	Caffeic acid, Ferulic acid
Others	Glycosides, carbohydrates, tannins

4.2.1 Anthocyanins: The Blue Pigment

The deep blue color of the butterfly pea flower is due to a group of acylated anthocyanins known as ternatins. These water-soluble pigments are notable for their pH sensitivity—turning red in acidic and greenish-yellow in alkaline conditions.

>Structure and Types:

Ternatins are derivatives of delphinidin and are acylated with glucose, p-coumaric acid, or malonic acid.

Ternatin	Color Contribution	Activity
Ternatin A1–F	Deep blue	Antioxidant, neuroprotective, natural colorant

> Applications

1. Natural Food Colorant

The blue anthocyanins (mainly ternatins) extracted from the petals are stable and safe natural pigments.

Used in confectionery, bakery, dairy products, beverages, and traditional sweets.

Advantage: Unlike synthetic dyes, they are non-toxic, biodegradable, and health-friendly.

Widely used in “butterfly pea tea”, a popular herbal drink that changes color with pH.

2. pH Indicator in Beverages

Anthocyanins from Clitoria ternatea are pH-sensitive:

Blue in neutral solutions

Reddish-purple in acidic solutions

Greenish-yellow in alkaline solutions

This property is applied in novel drinks and cocktails as a natural, safe "color-changing" agent.

3. Antioxidant and Health Benefits

Anthocyanins act as potent antioxidants, protecting cells from oxidative stress.

Reported benefits include:

Anti-inflammatory and anti-obesity effects

Neuroprotection (enhancing memory and cognitive functions)

Cardiovascular protection by reducing lipid peroxidation and improving vascular health

Contributes to the plant's use in Ayurveda and modern herbal medicine.

4. Cosmetic and Pharmaceutical Applications

Incorporated in natural skin-care products due to UV-protective and anti-aging properties.

Studied for their role in wound healing and anti-cancer research.

Potential for use in nutraceutical formulations (capsules, powders, functional foods).

5. Textile and Dyeing Industry

Used as an eco-friendly dye for fabrics and handicrafts.

Provides shades ranging from blue to purple, depending on mordants and pH of the dye bath.

Sustainable alternative to synthetic textile dyes.

6. Biotechnological Applications

Employed in biosensors due to their pH sensitivity and stability.

Studied for potential role in packaging materials (e.g., intelligent food packaging that changes color when food spoils).

4.2.2 Flavonoids

Flavonoids in Clitoria ternatea are responsible for its anti-inflammatory, cardioprotective, and antioxidant actions.

Flavonoid	Function
Kaempferol	Antioxidant, anti-cancer
Quercetin	Anti-inflammatory, anti-allergic
Myricetin	Antioxidant, neuroprotective

These compounds are primarily found in flowers and leaves.

4.2.3 Alkaloids

The major alkaloid identified is clitorine, which is thought to contribute to the plant's nootropic (memory-enhancing) and anxiolytic effects.

Found mainly in roots and seeds.

Shows moderate CNS activity in animal models.

Requires further clinical investigation for potential therapeutic use.

4.2.4 Triterpenoids and Saponins

Triterpenoids like taraxerol and taraxerone are known for their anti-inflammatory and hepatoprotective actions.

Saponins, particularly clitoriasides, possess:

Antimicrobial activity.

Hemolytic properties.

Immune-modulating effects.

They are primarily found in the roots and seeds.

4.2.5 Phenolic Compounds

Phenolics, such as caffeic acid and ferulic acid, are powerful free radical scavengers and play a key role in:

Skin protection

Anti-aging

Reducing oxidative stress

These compounds contribute to the plant's use in cosmetics and wellness supplements.

4.2.6 Other Identified Compounds

> Sterols

Beta-sitosterol: Anti-inflammatory, cholesterol-lowering properties

Found in leaves and roots.

> Carbohydrates and Amino Acids

Support nutritional value and energy supply

Contribute to the plant's tonic and restorative uses.

> Tannins

Present in leaves and seeds

Contribute to astringent and antimicrobial properties.

> Distribution of Compounds in Different Plant Parts

Plant Part	Major Constituents
Flowers	Ternatins, Flavonoids, Phenolics
Leaves	Flavonoids, Tannins, Saponins
Roots	Alkaloids, Triterpenoids, Sterols
Seeds	Alkaloids, Saponins, Proteins

4.3 Extraction Techniques

4.3.1 Solvents Used:

Water: Common for traditional teas, but limited in compound diversity.

Ethanol & Methanol: Extract a broader range of flavonoids and alkaloids.

Hydroalcoholic extracts: Offer a balanced profile of polar and non-polar compounds.

4.3.2 Extraction Methods:

1. Aqueous Extraction

Traditional method commonly used in herbal teas and ayurvedic preparations.

-Process:

> Fresh or dried petals are boiled or steeped in water.

> The filtrate is collected and concentrated.

Applications: Safe for food and beverage industry (e.g., butterfly pea tea).

Limitation: Lower pigment yield compared to organic solvents.

2. Solvent Extraction (Conventional Method)

Solvents used: Ethanol, methanol, acetone, or water (acidified with citric, acetic, or hydrochloric acid).

Steps:

> Dried petals are powdered.

> Powder is soaked/refluxed in acidified solvent.

> Extract is filtered, evaporated, and stored.

Advantages: High yield of anthocyanins and flavonoids.

Limitation: Toxicity issues if non-food grade solvents are used.

3. Ultrasound-Assisted Extraction (UAE)

Principle: High-frequency ultrasound waves disrupt cell walls, enhancing solvent penetration.

Benefits:

Faster extraction time.

Higher anthocyanin yield compared to conventional methods.

Uses less solvent.

Applications: Extraction of pigments for nutraceuticals and functional foods.

4. Microwave-Assisted Extraction (MAE)

Principle: Microwaves rapidly heat the plant matrix, releasing bioactive compounds.

Benefits:

Efficient and eco-friendly.

Reduces extraction time drastically.

Overheating may degrade anthocyanins.

5. Enzyme-Assisted Extraction (EAE)

Method: Enzymes such as pectinase and cellulase break down cell walls, releasing anthocyanins and other flavonoids.

Benefits:

Mild process preserving bioactivity.

Enhances extraction yield.

Limitations: Expensive enzymes, optimization needed.

6. Supercritical Fluid Extraction (SFE)

Method: Uses supercritical CO_2 with ethanol as a co-solvent.

Advantages:

Solvent-free, eco-friendly, high purity.

Selective extraction possible.

Limitations: High cost and technical expertise required.

7. Solid-Phase Extraction (SPE) & Purification

Use: To purify anthocyanins after initial extraction.

Method: Extracts are passed through C18 SPE columns, separating pigments from sugars, proteins, and other phenolics.

Produces highly purified anthocyanin fractions for pharmaceutical and analytical applications.

8. Stabilization of Extracts

Since anthocyanins are sensitive to pH, temperature, and light, stabilization is essential:

Acidification: Adding citric or tartaric acid.

Encapsulation: Using microencapsulation, spray drying, or liposomes.

Stabilizers: Sugars, ascorbic acid, or natural polymers.

Chapter 5: Pharmacological Activities

Clitoria ternatea has been a part of traditional medicine for centuries, especially in systems like Ayurveda, Siddha, and Unani.

In recent years, numerous preclinical and in vitro studies have validated its wide range of pharmacological activities.

These effects are largely attributed to its rich content of flavonoids, anthocyanins (ternatins), triterpenoids, saponins, and alkaloids.

> Nootropic (Memory-Enhancing) Activity

Clitoria ternatea is known in Ayurveda as a "Medhya Rasayana", i.e., a rejuvenator of the mind.

Key compounds: Clitorine, quercetin, ternatins.

Mechanism: Enhances cholinergic activity, increases acetylcholine levels, reduces oxidative damage to neurons.

Evidence: Animal studies show improvement in learning and memory in mice and rats using root and leaf extracts.

Modulates brain neurotransmitters (acetylcholine, dopamine).

Potential candidate for treating Alzheimer's disease.

> Antioxidant Activity

Due to its high anthocyanin (ternatin) and flavonoid content, the plant exhibits strong free radical scavenging abilities.

Mechanism: Inhibits lipid peroxidation, reduces reactive oxygen species (ROS).

Test models: DPPH, ABTS, and FRAP assays.

Phytochemicals involved: Ternatins, quercetin, kaempferol, phenolic acids.

Applications:

Anti-aging products

Cardiovascular protection

Neuroprotection

> Anti-Inflammatory Activity

Extracts tested: Ethanol and aqueous extracts of root and leaves.

Models used: Carrageenan-induced paw edema in rats.

Findings: Comparable anti-inflammatory activity to standard NSAIDs.

Mechanism: Inhibition of prostaglandin synthesis and inflammatory cytokines.

Compounds responsible: Taraxerol, flavonoids.

> Antimicrobial Activity

Clitoria ternatea exhibits activity against bacteria, fungi, and protozoa.

Bacteria inhibited:

Staphylococcus aureus

Escherichia coli

Pseudomonas aeruginosa

Bacillus subtilis

Fungal strains:

Candida albicans, Aspergillus niger

Mechanism: Disrupts microbial cell walls and interferes with DNA replication.

Compounds involved: Saponins, flavonoids, tannins.

Applications: Herbal sanitizers, toothpaste, and natural preservatives.

> Anti-Diabetic Activity

The plant has shown glucose-lowering effects in various experimental models.

Tested on: Alloxan and streptozotocin-induced diabetic rats.

Mechanism:

Increases insulin secretion.

Enhances glucose uptake in peripheral tissues.

Reduces blood glucose and HbA1c levels.

Active compounds: Flavonoids, alkaloids, phenolic acids.

Potential Use: As a natural adjunct in diabetes management.

> Anti-Cancer and Cytotoxic Activity

Though still in early stages, in vitro studies show cytotoxic effects of Clitoria ternatea extracts on cancer cell lines.

Affected cell lines:

Breast cancer (MCF-7)

Colon cancer (HCT-116)

Cervical cancer (HeLa)

Mechanism: Induction of apoptosis, inhibition of cell proliferation, DNA damage.

Key compounds: Ternatins, flavonoids, saponins.

> Anxiolytic and Antidepressant Activity

Animal models have demonstrated anti-anxiety and antidepressant effects of Clitoria ternatea.

Mechanism:

Modulation of serotonin and dopamine levels.

Inhibition of monoamine oxidase (MAO).

Tests used: Elevated plus maze, forced swim test, tail suspension test.

Extracts: Methanolic and aqueous extracts of roots and leaves.

Implication: Potential herbal remedy for stress, depression, and anxiety disorders.

> Hepatoprotective Activity

Models used: Carbon tetrachloride (CCl_4)-induced liver toxicity in rats.

Findings: Reduction in liver enzymes (ALT, AST, ALP), improved histopathology.

Mechanism: Antioxidant defense, membrane stabilization.

Parts used: Root and flower extracts.

> Anti-Asthmatic and Bronchodilator Activity

Traditionally used to treat asthma and bronchitis, scientific studies confirm bronchodilatory effects.

Extracts: Ethanolic extracts of roots and seeds.

Activity: Relaxation of tracheal smooth muscles.

Mechanism: Histamine receptor antagonism, anti-inflammatory effects.

> Anti-Ulcer Activity

Extracts of Clitoria ternatea have demonstrated protective effects against gastric ulcers.

Models: Aspirin and alcohol-induced ulcers in rats.

Mechanism: Enhances mucus production, reduces gastric acid secretion.

Effectiveness: Comparable to standard drugs like omeprazole in some studies.

> Diuretic and Antipyretic Activities

Diuretic: Increases urine volume and electrolyte excretion.

Antipyretic: Reduces fever induced by yeast injection in rats.

Application: Useful in managing fluid retention and fever naturally.

> Wound Healing Activity

Topical application of leaf or root paste accelerates wound contraction and epithelialization.

Mechanism: Stimulates fibroblast activity and collagen synthesis.

Models: Excision and incision wound models in rats.

Formulations: Used in herbal ointments and gels.

> Other Reported Activities

Activity	Notes
Anti-convulsant	Delay in onset and reduction of seizures
Anti-fertility (in males)	Suppressive effect on sperm count (in high doses)
Insecticidal	Toxic to mosquito larvae and some pests
Anthelmintic	Effective against intestinal worms in animals

Chapter 6: Traditional and Ethnomedicinal Uses

For centuries, Clitoria ternatea has been revered in various traditional systems of medicine including Ayurveda, Siddha, Unani, and Traditional Chinese Medicine. Known by names such as Aparajita in Sanskrit and Gokarna in Hindi and Marathi, the plant has been widely used by indigenous communities for treating numerous ailments ranging from neurological disorders to skin diseases.

This chapter explores the ethnomedicinal applications of Clitoria ternatea, categorized by medical system, plant part used, and therapeutic purpose.

6.1 Use in Ayurveda, Siddha, Unani

> In Ayurveda

In Ayurveda Clitoria ternatea is classified as a "Medhya Rasayana"—a group of rejuvenating herbs that enhance intellect, memory, and cognitive function.

Ayurvedic Properties	Details
Rasa (Taste)	Tikta (bitter), Kashaya (astringent)
Guna (Quality)	Laghu (light), Ruksha (dry)
Virya (Potency)	Sheeta (cold)
Vipaka (Post-digestive effect)	Katu (pungent)
Dosha Effect	Pacifies Pitta and Kapha

Common Ayurvedic Uses:

Shankhpushpi substitute: For enhancing memory and concentration.

Aparajita churna: Root powder used as a nervine tonic.

Kashayam (decoction): For treating fever, infections, and urinary tract issues.

Nasya therapy: Root juice instilled in nostrils for sinus and epilepsy.

> In Siddha: Known as Sangu Poo

Used for treating:

Eye infections (infusions)

Male infertility (seed extract)

Poison bites and skin boils (paste application)

> In Unani:

Used as Muqawwi-e-Asab (nerve tonic) and Muhallil-e-Waram (anti-inflammatory agent)

Prescribed for:

Epilepsy

Stress and anxiety

Swelling and abscesses

6.2 Folk and Tribal Medicine

Across tribal and rural communities in India, Southeast Asia, and Africa, Clitoria ternatea is considered a sacred and medicinal plant.

Use	Plant Part	Mode of Administration
Snakebite and scorpion sting	Root	Paste applied to wound; juice taken orally
Fever and body ache	Leaves and flowers	Decoction consumed twice daily
Infertility and low libido	Seeds and root	Powder mixed with milk or ghee
Menstrual irregularities	Root and leaf paste	Applied externally or taken as tea
Wound healing	Leaves	Poultice applied to affected area
Cough and asthma	Roots	Boiled in water; taken as herbal tea

6.3 Spiritual and Ritualistic Uses

The white-flowered variety is considered highly auspicious in Hinduism.

Flowers are offered to Goddess Durga and Lord Shiva during rituals.

In rural traditions, it is believed that keeping Clitoria ternatea near the home wards off negative energy.

Used in Pooja ceremonies as a symbol of victory and purity.

Known as "Aparajita" (meaning "undefeated") symbolizing divine strength.

6.4 Traditional Preparations

1. Aparajita Root Powder (Churna)

Ingredients: Dried roots.

Method: Powdered finely and taken with honey or milk.

Indication: Memory enhancement, anxiety relief, fever.

2. Flower Infusion (Tea)

Ingredients: Fresh or dried blue flowers.

Method: Steeped in hot water for 5–10 minutes.

Optional Additives: Lemon juice (for color change), honey.

Indication: Antioxidant, stress reliever, digestive aid.

3. Paste Application

Ingredients: Fresh leaves or roots.

Method: Ground into a paste.

Use: Applied to wounds, insect bites, and boils.

4. Kashayam (Decoction)

Boiled extract of roots and leaves.

Taken for fevers, respiratory problems, and urinary tract infections.

6.5 Comparison with Other Medhya Herbs

Clitoria ternatea is often compared to other cognitive enhancers like:

Herb	Common Use	Comparison
Shankhpushpi (Convolvulus pluricaulis)	Memory, stress relief	Similar CNS effects, but different plant family
Brahmi (Bacopa monnieri)	Neuroprotection	Works synergistically with Clitoria
Mandukaparni (Centella asiatica)	Learning and mental clarity	Combined use seen in classical formulations

These herbs are sometimes used together for enhanced nootropic effects in traditional medicine.

6.6 Safety and Precaution in Traditional Use

Traditionally regarded as safe in moderate doses.

High doses of seed extract may have anti-fertility effects (used traditionally for male contraception).

Some tribes caution use during pregnancy.

Always combined with adjuvants like milk, ghee, or honey to balance its potency.

6.7 Continuity into Modern Herbal Practice

The traditional uses of Clitoria ternatea continue to influence modern:

Ayurvedic formulations (e.g., Medhya Rasayana churna).

Herbal teas and infusions marketed for cognitive wellness.

Skin and hair care products incorporating flower extract.

Alternative treatments for stress, insomnia, and fatigue.

Chapter 7: Modern Applications

With a resurgence of interest in plant-based therapeutics, Clitoria ternatea has become a focus of modern research and product development. Thanks to its rich phytochemical profile and historical medicinal use, this plant is now widely utilized in pharmaceuticals, nutraceuticals, cosmetics, food products, and scientific research.

This chapter explores the diverse modern applications of Clitoria ternatea, highlighting its integration into contemporary health, beauty, and food industries.

7.1 Pharmaceutical and Therapeutic Applications

Pharmaceutical industries are investigating Clitoria ternatea as a source of bioactive compounds for use in:

1. Cognitive Health Formulations:

Used in herbal capsules, syrups, and tonics for:

Memory enhancement.

ADHD and age-related cognitive decline.

Stress and insomnia.

Commonly paired with Brahmi and Ashwagandha in Ayurvedic products.

2. Antioxidant Supplements:

Extracts used in anti-aging and free-radical defense supplements.

Marketed as a natural remedy for:

Neurodegeneration.

Cardiovascular health.

General immunity boosting.

3. Adjunct in Diabetes and Hypertension Management:

Found in sugar-control herbal teas and tablets.

Exhibits potential as an add-on therapy for:

Lowering blood glucose.

Improving lipid profile.

Reducing oxidative stress in metabolic syndrome.

4. Antimicrobial Products:

Incorporated into:

Herbal mouthwashes.

Toothpastes.

Sanitizers.

Effective against oral and skin bacteria.

7.2 Nutraceuticals and Functional Foods

The flowers and leaves of Clitoria ternatea are rich in anthocyanins, which make them popular in:

1. Herbal Teas: Known as "Blue Tea"

Promotes:

Detoxification.

Weight management.

Relaxation and sleep.

Often marketed as caffeine-free with mood-lifting properties.

2. Color-Changing Beverages

The tea changes color based on pH:

Blue (neutral).

Purple (with lemon or acid).

Used in cocktails, mocktails, and smoothies.

3. Natural Food Coloring

Ternatin pigments used in:

Baked goods.

Ice creams and desserts.

Rice and noodles in Southeast Asia.

4. Health Drinks and Tonics

Added to beverages aimed at enhancing:

Brain function.

Vision clarity.

Energy levels.

7.3 Cosmetic and Personal Care Products

With increasing demand for clean beauty and plant-based skincare, Clitoria ternatea is now featured in:

1. Hair Care

Found in: Hair oils, Shampoos, Serums.

Benefits:

Strengthens roots.

Reduces hair fall.

Promotes scalp health.

2. Skincare

Antioxidant and anti-inflammatory action useful in:

Anti-aging creams.

Face masks and scrubs.

Under-eye treatments.

3. Color Cosmetics

Used as a natural dye in:

Lip and cheek tints.

Organic eye shadows.

4. Soap and Bath Products

Flower extract infused in soaps for a cooling and calming effect on skin.

7.4 Agricultural and Veterinary Applications

1. Green Manure and Soil Enrichment

Clitoria ternatea is a nitrogen-fixing legume.

Used to improve:

Soil fertility.

Crop yield.

Sustainable farming practices.

2. Fodder Crop

Nutritious leaves and seeds used as cattle and goat feed.

Increases milk yield and animal health.

3. Natural Pesticide/Insect Repellent

Extracts tested for:

Mosquito larvicidal activity.

Crop protection.

Organic farming.

7.5 Industrial and Commercial Products

Product Type	Example Use
Herbal Supplements	Capsules for memory, stress relief, and vision
Functional Beverages	Blue tea blends, lemon flower tonics
Nutraceuticals	Powders and tablets with concentrated extracts
Natural Dyes	Food-grade coloring for confectionery and textiles
Cosmetics	Face serums, herbal soaps, shampoos
Eco-friendly Packaging	Bioplastic research using plant residue

7.6 Technological Innovations

Modern science has advanced Clitoria ternatea applications using technologies such as:

1. Nanoformulations

Nanoparticles from flower extracts tested for:

Drug delivery.

Antimicrobial coatings.

Enhanced antioxidant delivery.

2. Bioassays and Genetic Studies

Research on: Cloning of anthocyanin biosynthesis genes.

Development of genetically engineered crops for better pigment yield.

3. Biosensors

Flower pigments used in pH-sensitive biosensor development.

7.7 Commercial Brands Using Clitoria ternatea

Some popular brands/products:

> Blue Tea India – Herbal infusions.

> Brew Blue – pH-changing cocktails and beverages.

> Just Herbs – Skin and hair products with Aparajita extract.

> Amrutam – Ayurvedic brain tonic using Clitoria ternatea.

> Organic India – Nootropic formulations and blue tea range.

7.8 Market Potential

The global herbal supplement market is projected to grow at 6–8% annually.Clitoria ternatea-based products have gained demand in:

India

Thailand

United States

Australia

Europe

With increasing awareness of natural wellness, the plant's versatility provides enormous scope for sustainable businesses and health innovation.

Chapter 8: Recent Research and Scientific Studies

Over the last two decades, Clitoria ternatea has been the subject of intense scientific investigation across disciplines such as pharmacology, biotechnology, neuroscience, and phytochemistry. Modern researchers are now validating what traditional systems have known for centuries — this plant possesses diverse therapeutic and industrial potential.

This chapter highlights recent scientific studies that explore the plant's pharmacological actions, active compounds, mechanisms of action, and potential future applications.

8.1 Areas of Active Research

Field Focus:

Pharmacology :- CNS effects, anti-diabetic, anti-inflammatory, anti-cancer properties.

Phytochemistry :-Identification of flavonoids, anthocyanins, alkaloids, and saponins.

Molecular Biology :- Gene expression in biosynthesis of blue pigments.

Biotechnology :- Use in nanotechnology, bioplastics, and biosensors.

Agriculture :- Soil enrichment, pest control, fodder potential.

8.2 Phytochemical Studies

Numerous studies have confirmed the presence of bioactive constituents, including:

Ternatins (anthocyanins): Water-soluble pigments responsible for blue color; potent antioxidants.

Flavonoids: Kaempferol, quercetin (anti-inflammatory, neuroprotective).

Saponins: Immunomodulatory and anti-fertility effects.

Alkaloids and Glycosides: Support nervous system and cardiovascular health.

Phenolic compounds: Free radical scavenging properties.

8.3 Neuropharmacological Research

One of the most promising areas is its effect on the central nervous system (CNS).

> Memory and Learning Enhancement

Extracts from roots and flowers improved memory retention in rats using the Morris Water Maze test.

Compared favorably with standard nootropic drugs like Piracetam.

> Antidepressant and Anxiolytic Effects

Alcoholic extracts showed:

Increased serotonin levels in animal models.

Reduced symptoms of depression and anxiety.

> Anti-epileptic Activity

Methanolic root extract delayed onset and reduced severity of seizures induced by pentylenetetrazole.

8.4 Anti-diabetic and Metabolic Effects

Aqueous flower extract demonstrated α-glucosidase and α-amylase inhibition → reducing postprandial blood glucose.

Lowered blood glucose and improved insulin sensitivity in diabetic rat models

Supporting study:

> BMC Complementary Medicine and Therapies (2020) – Demonstrated dose-dependent hypoglycemic effects.

8.5 Anti-inflammatory and Analgesic Properties

Ethanol extracts reduced paw edema and inflammation in rats.

Significant analgesic effects in hot plate and tail-flick tests.

Mechanism: Inhibition of COX-2 and prostaglandin synthesis.

8.6 Anticancer Potential

Preliminary in vitro studies show promise in:

Cell Line	Effect
Breast cancer (MCF-7)	Cytotoxicity and apoptosis induction
Colon cancer (HT-29)	Cell cycle arrest
Liver cancer (HepG2)	ROS-mediated cell death

Compounds involved: Kaempferol, ternatins, and cyclotides

Research highlight:

> Journal of Natural Products (2019) – "Cytotoxic activity of blue pea flower anthocyanins in cancer cell lines"

8.7 Antioxidant and Anti-aging Studies

High ORAC (Oxygen Radical Absorbance Capacity) score.

Prevents oxidative DNA damage and lipid peroxidation.

Commonly used in anti-aging skincare research.

8.8 Antimicrobial and Antiviral Activity

Effective against Staphylococcus aureus, E. coli, Candida albicans.

Potential antiviral action reported against herpes simplex virus (HSV) and influenza virus.

Mechanism: Disruption of microbial cell walls and inhibition of protein synthesis.

8.9 Research in Nanotechnology

Silver nanoparticles synthesized using Clitoria ternatea extract:

Showed enhanced antimicrobial activity.

Explored for drug delivery and biosensing.

Example:

> Applied Nanoscience (2021) – "Green synthesis of AgNPs using Clitoria ternatea and its biomedical applications".

8.10 Research Gaps and Limitations

Despite growing evidence, key limitations exist:

Most studies are in vitro or animal-based.

Lack of long-term human clinical trials.

Dosage standardization is needed for safety and efficacy.

Pharmacokinetics and toxicity data are incomplete.

8.11 Ongoing and Future Research Areas

Clinical trials on cognitive disorders and depression.

Biotech applications for sustainable dye production.

Studies on fertility modulation and reproductive health.

Formulation development for functional food and pharma products.

Gene expression profiling of anthocyanin-producing pathways.

Chapter 9: Conservation and Sustainable Use

As interest in Clitoria ternatea continues to grow for its medicinal, agricultural, and commercial applications, it becomes essential to ensure that its cultivation, harvesting, and use are conducted in a sustainable and ecologically responsible manner.

Conservation is not just about protecting a species but also about maintaining biodiversity, ensuring fair access, and preserving traditional knowledge for future generations.

9.1 Importance of Conservation

Biodiversity Preservation: Clitoria ternatea is part of diverse ecosystems and plays a role in pollination and nitrogen fixation.

Genetic Diversity: Protecting different landraces and wild varieties ensures resilience against climate change and disease.

Cultural Significance: Used in Ayurveda, Siddha, Unani, and folk traditions; conserving it also protects ethnomedicinal heritage.

Rising Demand: Its increasing use in cosmetics, herbal teas, supplements, and research may lead to overexploitation if not managed properly.

9.2 Threats to Sustainability

Threat	Description
Overharvesting	Wild populations are reduced due to unregulated collection.

Habitat destruction	Deforestation, urbanization, and land use changes.
Poor cultivation practices	Use of pesticides, monocropping, and poor soil management.
Loss of traditional knowledge	Younger generations are less involved in ethnobotany.
Climate change	Alters flowering time, seed viability, and pest incidence.

9.3 In-Situ & Ex-Situ Conservation Strategies

> In-situ conservation involves protecting the plant in its natural habitat.

Establishment of herbal gardens and botanical reserves.

Community-led protection of wild-growing populations.

Sacred groves and traditional conservation zones used by tribal communities.

Agroforestry integration: growing Clitoria ternatea alongside other medicinal species.

> Ex-situ conservation is done outside natural habitats, using controlled environments.

Seed banks (e.g., ICAR-NBPGR): Store seeds for genetic preservation.

Botanical gardens: Preserve live specimens.

Tissue culture and micropropagation: Mass-produce genetically stable clones for reforestation or study.

DNA barcoding: For identification and classification of various strains.

9.4 Sustainable Harvesting Practices

To maintain Clitoria ternatea populations, wild or cultivated, harvesting must be eco-conscious.

Practice	Description
Selective Harvesting	Only mature flowers and pods are harvested.
Rotational Harvesting	Allows rest periods for plant regrowth.
Post-harvest care	Leaving part of the plant to ensure reseeding.
Community Training	Educating local collectors on best practices.
Avoid uprooting	Unless for propagation or necessary research.

9.5 Organic and Eco-friendly Cultivation

The cultivation of Clitoria ternatea in an organic and eco-friendly manner emphasizes harmony with nature while maintaining soil fertility and biodiversity. This perennial leguminous climber is well adapted to tropical and subtropical climates, where moderate rainfall and temperatures between 20–35 °C support its growth. The crop performs best in well-drained sandy loam to loamy soils with a neutral to slightly acidic pH. To prepare the land, farmers usually plough two to three times to achieve a fine tilth and then enrich the soil with organic manures such as farmyard manure, vermicompost, or green leaf manure. These natural amendments not only improve soil structure but also enhance microbial activity, which plays a vital role in nutrient cycling. Neem cake or mustard cake may also be incorporated into the soil, serving the dual purpose of providing nutrition and acting as a natural repellent against soil-borne pests.

In organic systems, seed selection is crucial. Farmers prefer locally adapted, non-hybrid seeds that have not been chemically treated. To improve germination and protect against fungal infections, seeds are often inoculated with biofertilizers such as Rhizobium, Azospirillum, or Trichoderma viride. Sowing is typically done at the onset of the monsoon under rainfed conditions, while irrigated fields allow year-round cultivation. Seeds are sown at shallow depths, and adequate spacing is maintained to ensure good air circulation and reduce disease incidence.

Nutrient management is achieved entirely through organic sources. Basal doses of compost and farmyard manure provide essential macronutrients, while biofertilizers enhance nitrogen fixation and phosphate solubilization. Foliar sprays of liquid manures such as Panchagavya or Jeevamrut are commonly applied at regular intervals, stimulating vegetative growth and improving flower production. Irrigation is applied judiciously, with emphasis on water conservation practices such as mulching, which helps retain soil moisture, suppress weeds, and regulate temperature around the root zone.

Weed management in organic cultivation avoids synthetic herbicides. Instead, manual weeding, mulching with crop residues, and intercropping with compatible legumes are adopted to minimize weed competition. Pest and disease control is likewise achieved using eco-friendly techniques such as spraying neem oil, cow urine extracts, or garlic–chilli decoctions. Natural enemies like ladybird beetles and predatory spiders are conserved by avoiding chemical pesticides, thus ensuring biological balance in the ecosystem.

Harvesting of flowers is usually done in the morning hours to preserve color and phytochemical content. Being a perennial plant, Clitoria ternatea continues to flower for several years if managed properly. The cultivation system, being organic, not only ensures sustainable yields but also maintains the medicinal and nutraceutical quality of the flowers and roots, which are widely used in Ayurveda and modern herbal industries.

Thus, organic and eco-friendly cultivation of Clitoria ternatea integrates soil health, biodiversity conservation, and safe pest management practices, making it a model medicinal plant for sustainable agriculture.

9.6 Role of Farmers and Local Communities

1. Custodians of Indigenous Knowledge:

Farmers preserve traditional wisdom about cultivation, seed selection, and eco-friendly practices.

Knowledge of medicinal and cultural uses is passed down generations.

2. Seed Conservation and Exchange:

Local communities maintain and exchange seeds of locally adapted varieties.

Ensures biodiversity and reduces dependence on commercial seed suppliers.

3. Organic and Sustainable Cultivation:

Adoption of organic manures, biofertilizers, and botanical pest repellents.

Intercropping with cereals or pulses for natural nitrogen fixation.

4. Cultural and Traditional Uses:

Flowers used in religious rituals, festivals, and as a natural dye.

Traditional medicine prepared at the household level.

5. Community Participation in Processing:

Women's self-help groups and small-scale entrepreneurs prepare tea, powders, and natural colorants.

Adds value and creates rural employment.

6. Environmental Conservation:

Use of eco-friendly farming reduces chemical pollution.

Mulching, composting, and biodiversity-friendly practices improve soil health.

7. Collective Marketing and Income Generation:

Community cooperatives market dried flowers, seeds, and extracts.

Provides an alternative income source for farmers.

8. Promotion of Local Economy:

Increases livelihood opportunities in rural areas.

Enhances self-reliance by linking traditional farming with modern herbal industries.

9.7 Institutional and Governmental Support

Several institutions and policies support the conservation of medicinal plants like Clitoria ternatea:

Organization/Policy	Role
National Medicinal Plants Board (NMPB)	Financial and technical support for cultivation and conservation
AYUSH Mission	Promotes sustainable herbal medicine use
ICAR & CSIR Labs	Genetic conservation and research

Tribal Welfare Departments	Integrating traditional knowledge and forest-based livelihood
Biodiversity Act, 2002	Recognizes rights of communities over plant genetic resources

9.8 Future Directions for Sustainable Use

1. Development of Eco-Friendly Cultivation Models:

Promote large-scale adoption of organic farming techniques.

Integrate with agroforestry and permaculture to conserve biodiversity.

2. Conservation of Genetic Diversity:

Establish seed banks and germplasm collections.

Encourage community seed-saving initiatives to protect indigenous varieties.

3. Value-Added Product Development:

Expand production of natural food colorants, herbal teas, nutraceuticals, and cosmetics.

Explore pharmaceutical formulations using bioactive compounds (e.g., anthocyanins, flavonoids).

4. Integration into Sustainable Farming Systems:

Promote intercropping with cereals and legumes to enhance soil fertility through nitrogen fixation.

Utilize Clitoria ternatea as a cover crop to prevent soil erosion.

5. Research on Pharmacological Properties:

Conduct advanced clinical trials to validate traditional medicinal claims.

Explore potential in neurological, anti-diabetic, antioxidant, and anticancer research.

6. Climate Resilience Studies:

Investigate adaptability of Clitoria ternatea under changing climatic conditions.

Breed improved varieties tolerant to drought, pests, and salinity.

7. Promotion of Community-Based Enterprises:

Support farmer cooperatives and women's self-help groups in processing and marketing.

Encourage fair-trade certification and organic labeling for better market value.

8. Awareness and Policy Support:

Integrate Clitoria ternatea into national medicinal plant conservation programs.

Provide subsidies, training, and incentives for sustainable cultivation.

9. International Trade Opportunities:

Position Clitoria ternatea as a natural, eco-friendly alternative to synthetic dyes and chemical supplements.

Strengthen India's role as a global supplier of herbal raw materials and value-added products.

10. Sustainable Use in Eco-Tourism and Landscaping:

Promote Clitoria ternatea as an ornamental and eco-tourism plant in botanical gardens and herbal parks.

Enhance public awareness of its ecological and cultural importance.

• References:-

1. Chakraborthy, G.S. Kumar, V. Gupta, S. et al. (2018). Phytochemical and Pharmacological Aspects of Clitoria ternatea – A Review. J. Appl. Pharm. Sci. Res.

> Open-access Indian journal, freely available online.

2. Tandey, R. Kumar, G.V. Sarkar, D. et al. (2024). In-Depth Review on Phytochemistry and Pharmacological Significance of Clitoria ternatea. J. Cardiovasc. Dis. Res.

> Indian journal, free access.

3. Tahseen, A. (2024). Pharmacological relevance of Clitoria ternatea (Aparajita): A review. J. Pharmacogn. Phytochem.

> Widely indexed Indian phytochemistry journal, easily downloadable.

4. Indian Herbal Pharmacopeia (IHPh), Vol I & II.

> Published by Indian Drug Manufacturers' Association (IDMA), contains Clitoria ternatea monographs.

5. Wealth of India – Raw Materials (CSIR, India).

> Classic reference on medicinal plants, includes Clitoria ternatea. Available in most Indian academic libraries.

6. Ayurvedic Pharmacopoeia of India (API).

> Govt. of India publication (AYUSH). Contains official data on Aparajita (Clitoria ternatea).

7. Kirtikar & Basu (Indian Medicinal Plants, 2 Vols).

> Traditional Indian text on medicinal plants, easily available.

8. Khare, C.P. (2007). Indian Medicinal Plants – An Illustrated Dictionary. Springer India.

> Covers botanical, pharmacological, and chemical info on Clitoria ternatea.

9. Nadkarni, K.M. (2007). Indian Materia Medica.

> Widely available Indian herbal medicine text.

➢ International Journals (accessible in India via open access or university subscriptions) :-

10. Athallah, D.R. et al. (2024). Pharmacological Potential of Butterfly Pea (Clitoria ternatea). Med. Prof. J. Lampung. (Open access).

11. Pham, T.N. et al. (2019). Extraction of anthocyanins from Butterfly pea flowers… IOP Conf. Ser.: Mater. Sci. Eng. (Open access).

12. Terahara, N. et al. (1990, 1996, 1998). Anthocyanins (Ternatins) from Clitoria ternatea. J. Nat. Prod./Tetrahedron Lett. (May need SciHub or library access).

13. Oguis, G.K. et al. (2019). Butterfly Pea, a cyclotide-bearing plant… Front. Plant Sci. (Free on PubMed/Frontiers).

14. Jeyaraj, E.J., Lim, Y.Y., Choo, W.S. (2022). Antioxidant, cytotoxic, and antibacterial activities of Clitoria ternatea flower extracts. Sci Rep. (Open access).